How To Get In Shape Fast

316 Great Fitness Tips For A Healthy Living

ADAM COLTON

Published by BizMove
www.bizmove.com

Disclaimer

All the content found in this book was created for informational purposes only. The Content is not intended to be a substitute for professional medical advice, diagnosis, or treatment. Always seek the advice of your physician or other qualified health provider with any questions you may have regarding a medical condition. Never disregard professional medical advice or delay in seeking it because of something you have read in this book.

316 Great Fitness Tips For A Healthy Living

There are many different reasons for starting up or intensifying your physical fitness program, but among the most popular are to enhance one's appearance, increase their overall level of health, and to prolong and improve the quality of their life. Use the information found in these tips to get started with your new plan.

1. One way to maximize your fitness routine is to join an online forum that deals with fitness. This will help in a number of ways that you might not have access to otherwise. You can get tips from pros, get ideas that you might not have come up on your own, attain a group sense of acceptance, have a way to brag about your workouts and show off what you have done.

2. Sex makes an amazing weight loss tool. This is some of the most exciting and least work-like exercise you can do. Healthy sex will help you get fit and is a great way to include your partner in your pursuit for weight loss. You will get in shape and improve your relationship.

3. Since getting regular exercise is essential when aiming to live a healthier lifestyle, you should try to find a workout buddy to exercise with you. Having a regular workout buddy keeps you motivated. You are much more likely to skip a workout if you are exercising on your own as opposed to having a workout buddy.

4. Swimming is a great way to get a full body workout. Swimming works out your arms when you use them to propel yourself forward in the water with strokes. It works out your legs as well when you kick them to balance your body in the water. You even use your core for balance and regulated breathing.

5. Pack a pair of comfortable shoes and a change of clothes in your car or briefcase. You'll always have the ability to switch out your dress clothes for clothes suitable for walking or perhaps even running. That way you can take the time to walk up the stairs instead of taking the elevator, walk to lunch instead of driving, and maybe even take a quick run.

6. When you are concentrating your fitness goals onto your abs, remember they need to rest. You will not do them any favors with daily workouts. You should limit your ab training to three days a week.

You should never do more than four days of ab training in a week.

7. By making a few minor modifications to your bench pressing routing, you can target different areas of the body. To focus on your chest muscles, try to squeeze the bar inward. You can switch the focus to your triceps by performing close-grip reps while squeezing the bar away from you or outward.

8. when in the gym, you can save more time by only resting when you need to. You shouldn't need to doing early sets as your muscles are just warming up. As your routines progress just rest as you need instead of wasting a set amount of time which you may not even need to use yet.

9. Before running a sprint race you should prepare by working on a faster stride. To help you increase speed, land your foot under your body not in front. Use your toes on the back leg to push off and move forward. Practice doing this and watch your running speed gradually increase.

10. A great fitness tip is to perform upright rows. Upright rows are a great exercise that can help develop your deltoids and your biceps. To correctly perform the upright row you'll want to grab the bar

at shoulder width. Then you'll want to lift your elbows up while keeping the bar close to your body.

11.   Do not be afraid to ask for help from a fitness trainer. They can give you recommendations on what foods to include in your diet, and they are available to cheer you on as you attempt to reach your fitness goals. They can also help you avoid common mistakes that people often make while working out.

12.   To build real strength, make sure you exercise your muscle groups in many different ways. Sticking with one form of exercise for a muscle group (like machine work only) can increase your strength in relation to that activity, but can actually weaken you when it comes to other activities that your body is not used to.

13.   Make exercise your morning habit. Set your alarm for a little bit earlier each morning, and try to perform some sort of physical exercise in that time frame. Eventually, your body will realize that this is when you wake up, this is what you will do, and it will grow to enjoy it.

14.   Satisfy your cravings. After a workout, your muscles will be craving proteins, but your brain will want sugar. Have them both to make sure you don't

sabotage your workout later with a binge. Limit your sugar intake to about twenty grams, as that should be enough to settle the cravings your body has.

15.   Some people are salty sweaters and will need to replenish their sodium levels during their exercise. If you notice white crust on your visor, your clothes or your skin, after your workout, you are someone who sweats out too much salt. Sodium can be replenished during your workout with pretzels and some sports drinks. If you feel like you sweat out too much salt, pay attention to any signs you may experience from low sodium, hyponatremia.

16.   Your neck can receive quite a bit of strain when doing crunches. Try to remember to place your tongue against the roof of the mouth while doing them. This should help with your head alignment and keep it properly set in place while minimizing the stress to the neck area.

17.   Make sure you are eating enough. Your body requires fuel. Your body especially requires fuel when you are working out. To keep in shape, you need to be getting the proper nutrition. Being fit does not mean eating less. If anything, you might find yourself eating more. Just make sure you are eating healthy.

18.   In order to maximize your fitness routine at the gym, be sure to only rest when needed between sets. This will save time, at the gym and get you moving to other activities quicker. Later on in your workout you'll need more rests, however you can start it off strong without any ill effects.

19.   Have a quick checkup done by a medical professional before you sign up for any scuba lessons. While learning to scuba dive can be a fun and exciting idea, make sure your lungs are in shape to handle it before you waste your money on something so pricey.

20.   In order to maximize your running fitness, be sure to give yourself a break every six weeks or so. This will allow your body to recover and help to prevent injury. During this break week, it is advisable to not rest completely, but to cut the workload in half.

21.   When choosing an exercise routine, choose something that you enjoy doing. If you enjoy doing the routine, chances are you will stick to it. If you dread your routine, you will continually make excuses as to why you can't or don't want to get in your workout for the day.

22.   A really good way to get fit is by enrolling in a cycling class. Most gyms typically offer cycling classes and they are a great way to get in shape and meet people. Instructors will push you and they usually play great music which makes the cycling more enjoyable.

23.   Choose the right shoes for your fitness program. The right shoe can make a difference in how far you run and how stable you are when you're lifting weights. Make sure you look for shoes later in the day when the food has widened. Make sure there is ample room to move your toes around and that there is a half-inch additional space for your big toe.

24.   Improving your strength is important while trying to get fit. Lifting heavy weights for shorter periods of time is better for the muscle and it will lessen the chance of getting muscle strain. This applies to running as well. Running harder for shorter periods, with breaks, will help you get stronger in a safe and healthy way.

25.   Add your favorite music to your workout. It has been proven that people who listen to music while working out go faster than those that aren't listening to music. Studies have also shown that people who listen to music while exercising perceive their workouts as being easier to complete.

26.   Most people don't realize that regularly performing dead lifts and squats can actually give your abdominal muscles a great workout as well. By performing at least five sets of ten reps each, your body is toned in a way that enhances your natural posture and firms the oblique muscles with no additional effort.

27.   Make sure to replace your workout shoes after a while to avoid having major knee injuries. It is generally suggested that you determine an expiration date of sorts on your workout shoes. To calculate this, figure that shoes generally last for about 500 miles. Take the number 500 and divide it by your weekly mileage to see how long your shoes should last.

28.   When you need shoes for working out, be sure that they fit properly. Go shoe shopping in the evening time. When it is late in the day, your feet are the largest. When trying on the shoes, be sure that you can wiggle your toes and that you have about a half inch of space between your longest toe and the shoe.

29.   Exercise during commercials. Long periods of television watching has been shown to encourage obesity. If you're going to watch television, you can

at least get moving during the commercial breaks. Do some light jogging up and down your stairs or skip rope for a few minutes until your program comes back on. This will help you to burn calories, even while doing something potentially unhealthy.

30.   Getting a punching bag or rubber human shaped punching target can provide an outlet for stress as well as a way to work on ones personal fitness. The punching will work out ones upper body including biceps, triceps, and deltoids. One will appreciate their punching bag the next time they need to let off some steam.

31.   If you are working on pull-ups, do not wrap your hand completely around the bar. The best method is to hook your thumb up by your index finger, as it will cause your arm muscles to work much harder to hold on to the bar. This also helps to improve your grip.

32.   When you are doing your working routine, try not to use a weight belt. Constantly using a weight belt can actually weaken the muscles in your lower back and abdominal muscles. Use it only when you are going to do maximal lifts in exercises including overhead press, deadlifts, and squats.

33.   To reach your fitness goals more quickly, follow this one tip : Move through mud. This means visualize yourself making all of your movements as if you were submerged in mud, try it. You'll see that you put much more effort into each movement and involve more muscles, increasing the burn more quickly, and thus, your improvement.

34.   If you are looking to get more fit, find a friend that will make the commitment to get in shape with you. With someone on your side, you will be held accountable for accomplishing your fitness goals. You can keep each other motivated and try new work out classes together. Finally, a friend can motivate you when you start slacking off.

35.   When working out some soreness is normal, but pain is not. Working out is often uncomfortable as you are working to increase your endurance and limits; however, it should not be outright painful. If you ever experience severe pain when working out, stop what you are doing immediately. If the pain does not subside, head to the doctor, as you may have suffered an injury.

36.   Add resistance training to your exercise plan. Resistance training helps build muscle. The more muscle you have in your body, the more quickly and efficiently you can burn calories. Resistance bands

or light weights are good options for working out at home. You can also use your own body weight to provide resistance. Exercises, such as push-ups and squats, make your muscles bear the weight of your body and that builds strength.

37.   Make sure you're not over doing your workouts. The best kind of workouts are those that push your body to its limit, but be careful not to go past your limit. You don't want to risk injuring yourself. Instead, start small and work your way up. A runner doesn't just jump into a 5k after not running for years, so you shouldn't either.

38.   Make sure you're stretching before and after your workouts. You want to do moving stretches, like jumping jacks and windmills, in the beginning, to loosen your muscles up. Afterwards, you should do stationary stretches to stretch out your muscles and let your body cool down, after your work out, to avoid getting any cramps.

39.   Swimming is an excellent low impact form of exercise that will help with weight loss. It will help you to burn calories, and get your body into shape. Swimming is also easier on people who have joint or muscle pain. When in the water you don't need to do a high impact workout, which can cause people pain.

40.   To keep your motivation going when it comes time to exercise, try paying your trainer in advance. With your hard-earned money in their hands, you should feel less likely to pull out of your workout session and feel more inclined to continue to see it through until you achieve your fitness goals.

41.   Instead of just doing as many crunches as you can, try doing some sit ups in your routine. Sit ups work your entire core and give you a better range of motion to work out, while crunches and other abdominal workouts, only target your abdominal muscles and not your core.

42.   Try to cut down the amount you rest during your time in the gym. Many people have limited time, and you should try and rest less during the beginning of your workout when your muscles are less tired, and at the end you can rest more when they are fatigued.

43.   Always cycle at a steady pace. By pedaling too quickly, you will become tired very fast. Pedal at a steady pace so that you do not become fatigued, and you build your endurance. Pedaling at a steady, but brisk pace can better inform you if you're close to injury since you'll most likely feel pulling.

44.   Building forearm strength is easier than you might know and can be done almost anywhere. When you are finished with your newspaper, save a few sheets for working out. Place a sheet from the paper on a table or other flat surface. Simply start at one corner and crumple it into your hand, pulling the paper in as you go. Try to make this take about 30 seconds for maximum effect. Do this with both hands.

45.   Slow and steady wins the race, the race to stay fit that is. A recent study showed that those who engaged in moderate physical activity, such as biking and walking, maintained the highest overall activity levels. Those who did vigorous exercises for short periods of time spent more of their day being sedentary. Vigorous exercise does burn calories, but those who enjoyed moderate exercise tended to be more active overall.

46.   When you are doing your working routine, try not to use a weight belt. Constantly using a weight belt can actually weaken the muscles in your lower back and abdominal muscles. Use it only when you are going to do maximal lifts in exercises including overhead press, deadlifts, and squats.

47.   Taking in lots of calcium can be great for certain fitness goals. Low-fat or skim milk is the best way

to get calcium without taking a lot of useless fat in with it. Calcium does not just build strong bones. Heavy doses of calcium improve the muscle-building process. Muscles grow stronger faster with plenty of calcium.

48.   To be more efficient with your workout time, try combining activities where possible. An example is using light weights to do some arm exercises while power walking on a treadmill. This works more muscle areas and burns more calories than doing each activity separately, great for working out on a schedule.

49.   Give different muscle groups a break. Working the same group of muscles, such as your abs, can become counterproductive if you don't give them some downtime to recover. Design your workout as a circuit of training that focuses on alternate areas of your body each day. This allows more recovery time and keeps your workouts more interesting.

50.   If you're looking to get in shape another thing to consider is to gradually increase the difficulty of your regimen. If you increase it too fast you will lose your motivation, and too slow, the results will be too slow. For example if you used to walk 30 minutes a day at a rate of three miles an hour

increase it to thirty minutes, or increase your speed to three and a half miles per hour.

51.   When you decide to get fit, take up running. Running is possibly the cheapest, most simple, most available fitness exercise in the world. Anyone can do it. While you can buy plenty of specialized gear for intense running programs, all you need to start with is a little research. Determine what sort of running is safe and effective for your current fitness level, and then hit the road!

52.   When trying to be physically fit, cardiovascular exercise should be a part of your fitness routine. Any type of movement that gets your heart beating fast (running, riding a bike) will help to burn calories, and keep off unwanted fat. Cardiovascular exercise will help keep your body healthy and strong.

53.   Bike riding is a wonderful past time for many americans. When they think of riding bikes, they think of wonderful memories from childhood. Riding a bicycle can also be a wonderful activity for any adult trying to lose weight. You will work up a sweat while on a bike ride, and be able to lose many calories-all while having a good time.

54.   Taking the proper supplements can assure that ones body is getting all the needed nutrients to improve fitness and refuel after exercising. Research should be done to decide what the best amounts for that individual will be. However with the right balance supplements will improve the results of exercising and increase overall fitness.

55.   Establishing a schedule that one will be able to follow and not conflict with other interests will ensure that one can dedicate themselves to their fitness. A schedule will enable one to keep track of what they have planned for themselves. Fitness will follow when one is following their routine.

56.   Strenuous workouts can put a great deal of strain on your muscles, especially in the neck area. To reduce tension and prevent strain when you do your sit-ups or crunches, hold your tongue on the roof of your mouth. This guarantees that your head and neck muscles are properly aligned in a natural position.

57.   Even if you sustain an injury to your right arm, don't avoid exercising your left arm. It is actually possible that by increasing the intensity of your left arm's workout, you may actually increase the strength in your injured arm by as much as ten percent over two weeks. By working out with your

uninjured arm, you are stimulating the nerve muscles of your injured arm.

58.   Make sure that you get the most out of your shoulder workouts. There are three parts that make up your deltoids and ideally, you want to hit all three, if you want a well developed muscle. Shoulder presses and lateral raises, are two of the best exercises you can do.

59.   A great fitness tip is to try doing bench presses at an angle. By changing the angle when you do your bench presses, you're putting emphasis on a different area of the muscle. Doing this can have significant results. You can either set the bench at an incline or a decline to change the angle.

60.   Be sure to include a balanced diet as part of your fitness routine. If you continue to eat unhealthy foods, you will never get the results that you want from your exercise program. Pay attention to the calories that you are eating as well; you want to make sure that you stay within the recommended daily limit.

61.   To build real strength, make sure you exercise your muscle groups in many different ways. Sticking with one form of exercise for a muscle group (like machine work only) can increase your strength in

relation to that activity, but can actually weaken you when it comes to other activities that your body is not used to.

62.   A healthy diet is an important part of any fitness program, and a daily serving of meat is essential for programs focused on building muscle mass. Meat is packed with protein, which makes the best fuel for muscle growth. Six to eight ounces of meat every day provides plenty of energy for growing muscles.

63.   Read up on how the body works. You will find it quite helpful when making diet and exercise decisions if you understand how the body works. Certain foods will digest faster than others and others will just basically turn to fat. Learning as much as possible will help in the long run.

64.   Stay limber by stretching often, and if you are getting older, hold your stretches for longer periods of time. Your muscles will remain warm, strong and loose, and you will be able to workout more vigorously. Stretching can also help reduce or prevent soreness of the muscles and increases flexibility.

65.   In order to achieve a physically fit body, it is important that you know how to repair you muscles fast. If this is done efficiently, you can be able to

workout your muscles as soon as they recover. Researchers found a fast way to repair muscles, and this is done by doing light exercises on the same muscles the following day.

66.   One way to maximize your fitness routine is to work out with a friend. This will help with positive thinking and also help to push you further than you might have gone otherwise. Humans typically are competitive in nature. This will add a sense of camaraderie and competition to your workouts.

67.   When starting a new exercise regime, have a plan! Make a list of your goals in an exercise journal. Choose a workout that you enjoy, and begin by performing a low intensity version of this. With each week, increase the intensity and add an extra five minutes to your workout. Remember to make a note of your progress in your exercise journal, as this will only encourage you to stick with the plan.

68.   Choose the ideal time of day for your body to exercise. A morning person will find it quite easy to fit in their workout routine early in the day, whereas someone who feels at their best later on in the day should wait until the afternoon or evening to exercise. If you work out when your body and mind is feeling in tip-top condition, you will get the best results possible.

69.   You can do some as much strength training as needed to meet your goals. If you want your muscles to look bigger, you should schedule less strength training reps. But if you're trying to chisel leaner, more sculpted muscles, then up the number of strength training workouts you get in.

70.   One basic tip for fitness is do not overtrain! Sometimes when you have a health or fitness goal you want to achieve, it is tempting to push yourself to your fullest capacity, but this is not healthy. Set regular achievable goals for yourself and results will be well within your reach.

71.   Avoid exercising when you are under the weather, unless you are only sick above the neck. To be on the safe side, it is best to just take the day off to rest. Besides that, all of your efforts from exercising would not go toward building your body up, but they'd go toward healing it from your illness.

72.   If you want your fitness program to succeed, surround yourself with other people who also make working out a priority. You will be motivated by their successes, and you can learn from their failures. Enthusiasm is often contagious; if your

friends and family members are excited about the results they are seeing, you will feel the same way.

73.   Make sure you get plenty of sleep. Sleeping is essential for all life. While you sleep, your body undergoes repairs that it could not normally do while you are awake. Your heart rate is also lowered, and you are in your most relaxed state. This is important when working out.

74.   A great way to get motivated once again if you are stuck in a rut in your fitness plan is to buy a new pair of gym shoes. Shopping always makes everyone feel good in general, but when you buy a new pair of gym shoes it's like getting a brand new tool to help you reach your fitness goals. You'll feel empowered as well as responsible for using great new shoes that you just spend your hard earned money on.

75.   Stepping classes are an especially great way for women to get fit. Stepping classes can shape up the thighs and butt, a region that's well-known for being important in feminine beauty! Other exercises such as body squats and lunges can also help to firm up these muscles as well. Trunk, core and thigh muscles are important to both genders, because they provide a majority of the body's lifting capability.

76. You can improve your fitness in less time each day by choosing exercises which do double duty. For example, while doing squats, do bicep curls using light weights, and while doing lunges, lift the weights straight up. To get the most out of each workout, be sure to concentrate on using proper form for both moves.

77. Find a way to sneak in exercise. It's not important where or when you exercise, just that you do exercise. It is easy to sneak in a thirty minute workout in your day. If you take a bus, get off a stop or two before your stop and walk the rest of the way or go for a walk after lunch. Finding small pockets of time to exercise can be beneficial to your health.

78. Video games are a great, fun way to get fit. There are lots of movement oriented games that will get you moving, such as Wii Fit and Dance Dance Revolution.

79. It is possible to stay active even during resting periods. You can lift some hand weights while watching television, or do some calf raises as you fold laundry.

80. Be careful with the types of supplements that you decide to take. While many of them may help if you use them correctly, when you aren't sure about the proper usage you can cause yourself either real physical damage or even mess up your fitness progress by ingesting too many calories.

81. If you are a newbie to the fitness world, then you should push your self to the point of pain and failure and then throw back a pint of supplement. It has been shown that people who do this gained over 5 pounds of muscle over just 8 weeks.

82. Design your fitness plan to avoid injury. This means using good posture and form while working out, using good equipment, and taking a rest day at least once a week. Replace your sneakers every few hundred miles to avoid leg injuries if you do a lot of walking or running.

83. Don't go for an all or nothing approach when it comes to fitness. Even if you can't fit in thirty minutes of exercise every day, that doesn't mean you shouldn't bother trying at all. Even if you can only get your thirty minutes in once a week, it's better than nothing. You can always work up to more workouts as time goes on.

84.   Once you have embarked on a new fitness routine, you may be tempted to overdo it. To build your strength and stamina, you should push yourself only slightly more each time you go into your chosen activity. Stretching afterwards is key to ensuring you protect the muscles you are building.

85.   When planning your exercise routine, put in resistance first and the aerobic exercise last. When exercising glycogen is used first and then fat is used for energy. Glycogen will be used for the energy for resistance exercises. Doing aerobic exercise next will help you to burn more fat because the stored glycogen has already been used.

86.   A great fitness tip you should add to your fitness regime is to build your forearm strength. This will help you tremendously when playing sports. One way you can achieve this is by crumpling up newspapers with each hand. Do this for around thirty seconds and eventually, you will notice a difference in your forearm strength.

87.   If you are about to start a new fitness regime and have not exercised before or in a long time, or have a medical condition of some sort that might be exacerbated by exercise, it is a good idea to see your doctor before you begin a program. Getting a

medical check up will help ensure that you choose the most beneficial exercise program for yourself.

88.   If you want to become better at hitting a softball, you should try playing Foosball. Foosball, also called table soccer, is a table game in which a ball is moved by controlling rods that are attached to player figurines. Playing Foosball on a regular basis will help you improve your hand-eye coordination, which will greatly assist you in hitting a softball.

89.   If you are an avid rock-climber, buy uncomfortably tight shoes. While this may seem counter-productive, it actually gives you the ability to feel every nook and cranny you may have otherwise missed, and your grip will be better. You should be able to stand in the shoes, but not walk in them.

90.   Motivate yourself in your own fitness goals by motivating others. You can have a huge impact on your own well being when you encourage someone else. It does not matter if it is a friend, or family member, you chose to build up. Improvement will breed improvement and you will both win.

91.   When working out, do so with a partner. Having a friend or family member with you when you work

out makes the time go faster and makes the
workout feel easier. It also takes the focus off the
discomfort or pain you are feeling during a
strenuous workout routine.

92.   When trying to gain muscles in your arms by
lifting weights, go light weights fast. It has been
proven that lifting light weights at a fast pace is just
as effective as lifting heavy weights at a slower pace.
You can try doing this method by using a bench
press and lifting weights that are 40 to 60 percent of
what you can handle. Push the weights up as fast as
you can.

93.   Before you get on the treadmill or the exercise
bike for the first time, make an appointment with
your doctor. The doctor's recommendations may be
critical, particularly for those for whom fitness is a
challenge. If you are relatively healthy already, your
doctor can assist you in getting the most of your
workouts.

94.   A great fitness tip is to make sure you assign the
appropriate amount of sets to each of your muscle
groups. You'll obviously want to perform more sets
for your chest than you would for your arms. This
is because your chest is a bigger muscle group than
your arms.

95.   You need to find a workout that you actually enjoy doing if you really want to be able to stick to it. If you do not like what you are doing it will be very difficult to find the motivation to do it on a regular basis. A lot of people make the mistake of thinking fitness has to be boring and repetitive when it does not have to be.

96.   Drink a lot of water throughout your day. The friction caused by muscle fibers moving past each other generates heat, which dehydrates your body. Your body uses sweat to cool the body and then it needs rehydrated.

97.   You can help to prevent knee injuries that can result from fitness by strengthening your hip muscles. This will help to lessen the burden on your knees, as your hips will have more control over the movement of your legs. Some simple exercises that can help to build hip muscles are lunges and bridges.

98.   Stretch after you workout. Most people know to warm-up before they start their workout. Less know that you need to stretch afterwards as well. Resist the urge to leave the gym or just sit down and relax once you're finished. Taking the time to stretch will keep you limber and maximize the effect of your workout.

99.   To increase your endurance, breathe fully and from your diaphragm when you exercise, particularly when running. This increases your oxygen intake and your lung capacity and lets you exercise longer. If you don't know how to breathe from your diaphragm, you can lie down and put something on your stomach, then practice making it rise and fall as you inhale and exhale.

100.   When you are running up hills, make sure to lean forward slightly, keep your head up and focus your eyes on the top of the hill. This helps to keep your airways open instead of closing them off as you would if you were hunched over. Keep your eyes on the goal ahead and you'll clear it in no time.

101.   Do not rely on a fitness routine that requires extensive equipment. Putting all of one's faith in equipment-intensive exercise leaves one at the mercy of the equipment. The savvy fitness enthusiast will have a varied exercise program that includes plenty of exercises that can be performed without equipment. These exercises prevent a breakdown of one's overall fitness strategy when equipment is temporarily unavailable.

102.   Diamond push ups are another push up modification that can be done to achieve greater

things you need to work on, and the extra time will translate to better results. Trouble areas won't be trouble too long if you give them special consideration.

117.   One should consider what they want to get from a gym before they pay for a membership. If one likes swimming then they should look for a gym with a pool. If one likes to run then they should look for a gym with a running track. Such important things can make big differences to how satisfied one is with their gym and actually go there to work on their fitness.

118.   Having a good friend or other person to work out with and improve fitness levels together will be beneficial to both people. They will have someone there to help spot them while working out. The other person can also help to increase motivation and give both individuals better fitness levels.

119.   No matter what your schedule is, make time for exercise. Now this doesn't mean that you have to be able to make it to the gym each and every day. Just make sure that you are getting some movement in every day, whether that's a walk at your lunch break, playing with the kids at the park or doing an exercise video before bed. Make a commitment to move your body every day.

120.   Even if you sustain an injury to your right arm, don't avoid exercising your left arm. It is actually possible that by increasing the intensity of your left arm's workout, you may actually increase the strength in your injured arm by as much as ten percent over two weeks. By working out with your uninjured arm, you are stimulating the nerve muscles of your injured arm.

121.   The longer you exercise, the more fat you will burn off at the gym. So, when you are working out at the gym or at home, make sure that you are listening to good music. Music should be uplifting, which can give you the motivation to push harder to reach your goal.

122.   Form is crucial in many of the exercises that you will be doing. Many people do not have the right form when they perform a squat. To do this, but a bench underneath you before you squat. Then bend your knees until your butt touches the bench.

123.   Giving a part of your home or your car a deep cleaning will not only improve the look of your house or vehicle, but burn a great deal of calories. Going to the gym or setting a time to exercise is not always necessary when you keep active and do high intensity activities.

124. To recover faster from heavy exercise, do a light work out the next day, that covers the same muscle group. On this second day, concentrate on very low weights, which are about twenty percent of your lifting capacity and two quick sets of twenty-five repetitions. Your muscles will heal faster because they will receive more blood and nutrients flowing through them.

125. Make your warm-up the same style of exercise as the one you will be strenuously performing. If you plan on running on a treadmill, you should first stretch, then walk slowly for a bit. Turn the slow walk into a brisk one, and you are ready for the run. You need to make sure the muscles are ready for the work.

126. Try creating a workout playlist. Start with some slower songs for your stretching and have them slowly get more fast paced. While you're working out you want good, fast paced songs to keep you moving. Then, you'll want the songs to slow down again for your cool down period.

127. A great fitness tip is to experiment with different set and rep ranges and see what works for you. Typically lower reps are better for building mass and strength. Higher reps are for muscle endurance.

A lot of sets can promote muscle gain but they can also lead to over training.

128.   To meet your fitness goals, keep an eye on your nutrition. If you want to get the full benefit of your workouts, don't forget to drink water and eat a balanced diet rich in protein, simple carbohydrates and complex carbohydrates. Calculate your daily caloric needs and keep track of your intake.

129.   Don't be afraid to ask for help at the gym. If you don't know how to use a machine, go ahead and ask. Understanding how to utilize both the aerobic and strength building machines will give you the confidence to actually use them. The more comfortable you are, the more likely you are to keep up your workouts.

130.   If you are going to be doing serious weight training, it is crucial to have a spotter on hand. As you are lifting, your body is going to get tired. Lifting without a spotter leaves you open to the danger of being unable to lift your weights off of your chest, or even more dangerously, having them fall down on you if your arms give out.

131.   A good tip to stay fit, is to try circuit training. Circuit training is a method of lifting weights where you dramatically reduce the rest time and the

weight. This method turns your weight lifting session into a cardio session at the same time, so you can kill two birds with one stone.

132.   Decrease your time in the gym by not taking as long to rest between sets of weightlifting. When you first begin lifting weights your muscles are still strong enough to go right through. Think intuitively and take breaks when you need them, but you can cut down a good 10-20% off your gym time by cutting down on those early breaks, which would allow you to move on to something else that much quicker.

133.   Diamond push ups are another push up modification that can be done to achieve greater fitness results than standard ones. To do them, simply place your hands on the floor and create a diamond shape. Then do push ups as you normally would. The closer your hands are to each other when in the diamond configuration, the harder it is to do.

134.   One of the biggest excuses not to exercise is that you have things to do. So why not buy a treadmill? Using a treadmill will allow you to get things done while you work. You can do school work, watch TV, go over your work assignments, or even just read a book.

135.   No matter which type of workout you choose to do, you need to stay hydrated. Drinking plenty of water before, during and after exercise helps to replace fluids that are lost during your workout. Staying hydrated means that you will have more energy to go that little bit further, and you will feel better overall.

136.   When you need shoes for working out, be sure that they fit properly. Go shoe shopping in the evening time. When it is late in the day, your feet are the largest. When trying on the shoes, be sure that you can wiggle your toes and that you have about a half inch of space between your longest toe and the shoe.

137.   When recovering from an injury, you should try and work out as soon as possible. Start out with only a few minutes here and there to test out if you are truly better. If you are, then you should start working out and build up the strength that you had lost while injured.

138.   Consider adding a few sit-ups to your crunch routines. Over the past few years sit-ups have been given a bad reputation. Be sure to avoid doing anchored-feet sit-ups. This particular variety of sit-ups can seriously strain your lower back.

139.   An elastic exercise band can be a good low resistance way for someone to work on their fitness. The bands also have the advantages of being highly portable so you can take them with you when you travel and use them in many different locations. An exercise band is another good fitness tool for someone to have.

140.   If you have jammed a finger playing sports or have a finger that often jams, tape it together with the finger that is next to it. By doing so, you strengthen the finger (two are stronger than one) and lessen the chance that it will turn in a strange angle while playing.

141.   If you injure one of your arms, don't stop exercising the opposite one. Technically, when you work out one of your arms the muscle nerves in the opposite arm are stimulated too. It's been found that working out one arm can increase the strength in the other by ten percent.

142.   Get into the habit of wearing a pedometer to help accomplish your fitness goals. You should be walking around 10,000 steps a day. If you are not up to that, increase your steps by 100 steps a day, or 500 steps a week, until you are regularly hitting the 10,000 mark.

143.   Pay attention to the toilet after your workout. Your urine color is the best indicator of being properly hydrated. Even if you are slightly dehydrated, it could make your exercise harder than it has to be. If you are hydrated your urine will be pale yellow with no strong odor, it should be this way before and at least an hour after your workout is finished. If your urine is dark, you need to drink more water while working out.

144.   Make sure to check your body for any signs of injury or disease. Go to your doctor regularly and have a check up and perform some tests with your doctor. This will ensure that you are keeping nice and healthy and nothing will pop up and surprise you

145.   Once you have embarked on a new fitness routine, you may be tempted to overdo it. To build your strength and stamina, you should push yourself only slightly more each time you go into your chosen activity. Stretching afterwards is key to ensuring you protect the muscles you are building.

146.   A good tip to stay fit, is to try circuit training. Circuit training is a method of lifting weights where you dramatically reduce the rest time and the weight. This method turns your weight lifting

session into a cardio session at the same time, so you can kill two birds with one stone.

147.   Talk a walk every evening. Walking is low impact and burns extra calories. It is a good way to start a work out routine for weight loss beginners. It is not only good for weight loss but it is also good for your general health and well being.

148.   Practice "Four-Square Breathing" after your workout while stretching. Breath in for four seconds, then breath out for four seconds, and repeat for three minutes. "Four-Square Breathing" increases your lung capacity and reduces stress when done properly, which helps you relax after your workout, and get ready for the rest of your day.

149.   There is always another option to get a workout in no matter how busy your life is. Are you dragging the kids to and from soccer practice? Why not get in your own walk or run while they are busy at practice. Do you love reading? Try downloading some audio books and going on a walk while listening to your favorite book.

150.   Arm lifts are a good way to give your arms a quick workout and to gain upper body strength. Simply take a chair, bed, table, or any elevated

surface that is the same height as your mid section when sitting down, and stand in front of it. Then take your arms and place them behind you on the surface. Crouch down a little until your arms bend into a 90 degree angle, and then rise up. Repeat 10 times for 3 sets.

151.   In order to build better abs, don't work your abdominal muscles too often. Your ab muscles are just like the other muscles in your body and require rest. Don't work your abdominal muscles two days in a row, only work them two or three days a week, with at least one day of rest in-between.

152.   Tackle the exercises you do not like by actually doing them. The rationale being that people are more inclined to avoid doing their weakest exercises. Add the one you do not excel at and practice it in your routine.

153.   If you have a gym membership, use every piece of equipment offered. Try not to use just one or two different exercise machines. Using a variety of machines will not only prove more fun, but you'll effectively work more parts of your body. Try to learn to use at least a dozen different machines in your gym.

154. If your workout program includes separate exercises for individual body and muscle groups, try this trick: After completing each set, take anywhere from twenty seconds to half a minute to stretch and flex the muscle you just targeted. Doing so may actually increase the strength of the muscle as much as 20 percent!

155. Work your hamstrings in order to make your sprint faster. Your hamstring muscles help your speed and are used to push off. Leg curl is a great exercise to get strong hamstrings, but instead of releasing this exercise quickly, release slowly which will work your hamstrings more. Strong hamstrings equal a faster sprint.

156. Strengthen your back to help end back pain. Every time you do a set of exercises that focus on your abdominal exercises, do a set of exercises that focus on your lower back. Working out only your abdominal muscles can cause poor posture and pain in the lower back.

157. Walk barefoot. This will help strengthen your calf muscles as well as your ankles. This is especially helpful for women, who shorten their calf muscles by walking in high heels so often. Stretching your leg and ankle muscles cuts down on stiffness and

encourages flexibility and mobility. Walking barefoot also helps your sense of balance.

158.   Your workouts should be under an hour if you are trying to grow muscle. If you exercise for over an hour, your body will produce more cortisol, a stress hormone, that can result in testosterone-blocking effect. It will also waste your muscle. The best way to avoid this is having short weight workouts.

159.   Exercise is great for any female experiencing PMS symptoms. It dose a variety of things that can ease the discomfort and pain associated with PMS. It can decrease bloating in the abdomen, promote weight loss which can also relieve many symptoms, help combat depression and anxiety caused by PMS, and reduce stress that PMS seems to make worse.

160.   Walking: We do it every day, but there's a good chance that we could be doing it a lot more. Even minor adjustments in your daily number of steps can contribute to weight loss. Try parking at the end of the lot, taking the stairs instead of the elevator, or simply taking a leisurely stroll around the block.

161.   If you aim to grow bigger and stronger, do not be afraid of meat. You should aim to eat around four to eight ounces on a daily basis in order to

effectively achieve these goals. Even though you can grow muscle without eating meat, studies have shown that people who ate meat gained much more muscle compared to people who did not.

162.   Shopping for new work-out clothes will boost your confidence and encourage you to meet your fitness goals. It may be something simple but you will want show people what you look like in it, at the gym!

163.   Finding a fitness buddy can motivate you to keep working out. By finding someone to work out with, you can have someone to talk to, hang out with, and hold yourself accountable to. You are less likely to skip out on a workout if you are supposed to meet someone there.

164.   Sit ups and push ups are really good tools to use for getting a lean body. The best thing about sit ups and push ups is that you can do them almost anywhere. You can do push ups and sit ups at almost any time of the day, all you need is a small window of time and you can execute a quick workout.

165.   When you are running up hills, make sure to lean forward slightly, keep your head up and focus your eyes on the top of the hill. This helps to keep

your airways open instead of closing them off as you would if you were hunched over. Keep your eyes on the goal ahead and you'll clear it in no time.

166.   Bench presses are a simple weighted exercise that you can do to work out your chest muscles. All gyms have bar weights for doing bench presses, but if you have one at home, you can do it there, or use dumb bells to replace a bar. Simply lay on your back on a weight platform and lift your arms into the air while holding the weight. Then lower your arms.

167.   One of the most effective ways to increase your swimming speed is to fully develop your ankles' flexibility. Think of your feet as flippers, which must be able to extend and flex as you propel yourself through the water. Before your water workout, sit down and grab your feet, flexing them away and from your body and holding each position for one minute.

168.   Use light exercise to recover from a hard muscle workout the day prior. Make sure you are exercising the same muscles as you did the day prior. Light weight is about 20% of what you originally used for lifting at one time. Use these light weights to do two sets of 25 repetitions to create more blood flow to repair your hurt muscles.

169.   To build more muscle, try multiplying what the overall weight you lift is by how many times you actually lift it. The great things is that there is a lot you can do to improve this number. You can try lifting more weight, doing more sets per routine, or doing more repetitions in each set.

170.   When using a work out bench you are not familiar with for the first time, you should test to make sure the padding is up to your specifications. Using your thumb, press into the seat to check the padding. If you feel wood or metal, find another weight bench.

171.   A great workout tip is to perform dips. Dips can work out both your triceps and your chest. To hit the triceps you should do dips with elbows in and your body straight. To hit the chest you should lean forward and flare your elbows out. You will feel a great pump at the end.

172.   Don't overcompensate for exercise by eating more food, or you will simply end up taking in excess calories. While exercise does increase your nutritional needs, the increase is not noticeably large. You don't need to make a conscious effort to increase your food intake unless you are working out for several hours a day.

173.   Do not be afraid to add unconventional workout programs to your fitness routine. If you want to jump rope or learn to tap dance, go for it! As long as you are staying active, there is no right or wrong way to work out. If you can make it fun, you are more likely to continue your quest for physical fitness. So, look around and see if you can find any classes or programs that you are interested in.

174.   Archery can be a way for one to work on their fitness while having fun and learning a new skill at the same time. The repetitive drawing of the bow's string will work ones upper body. Drawing with each arm will ensure that both sides get exercise. The walking to retrieve arrows will also has fitness benefits.

175.   Ankle flexibility is a key focus for development when swimming. You can swim faster and more effectively by increasing your "flipper" capability in your feet. Seat yourself on the ground; shoes off. Extend your legs to the front with heels firm on the ground and then simply point forward with your toes as far as you can, then point them back towards your shins. About 1 minute a day will do the trick.

176.   Stretch appropriately to prevent muscle strain and injury. The right amount of time to stretch

depends on your age. Hold stretches for 30 seconds if you are younger than 40 years old, and hold them for 40 seconds if you are above 40. Muscles grow less pliable with age. A decline in muscle pliability usually occurs past the age of 40, requiring you to stretch longer to stay limber and injury free.

177.   Even though it is vital, sleep is often overlooked when one plans a fitness regimen. The modern world tends to encourage one to sleep less and less. This is a mistake if one wants to get fit. Sleep is crucial in restoring the body and maintaining energy levels. Get at least seven hours of sleep every night to stay fit and healthy.

178.   Jumping rope is usually associated with children but it is actually an ideal " and fun - way to lose weight and improve your health. Jumping rope is a cardiovascular exercise that can also tone your muscles. It gets your heart pumping, burns calories and works out your entire body. Make sure you jump on an exercise mat or a wood floor to reduce the impact on your ankles and knees. Carpeting is soft, but it's very easy to twist your ankle on this surface when wearing running shoes. Research has also found that jumping rope over the course of many years can help to prevent osteoporosis, so grab that rope and start jumping your way to a thinner, healthier you.

179.   Determine what you are trying to accomplish with your workouts and write it down. Maybe you are trying to lose weight, gain strength, or just stay young longer. Writing down what you are doing and why will help you stay motivated and help you pinpoint items that you need to focus on.

180.   You need a strong core. If your core is strong and stable, it will help you with every exercise that you do. Sit-ups are a classic exercise and one that builds the core muscles. Doing sit ups can also increase the range of motion you experience. Stronger abs are able to work longer and harder.

181.   Fit in some stretching exercises when you are sitting at your desk at work. It is not good for your body when you sit at your desk for hours without getting up. Every 60 to 90 minutes, if you can get up and stretch for five minutes, you can increase the circulation in your muscles and prevent muscle cramps.

182.   A different way to exercise and maintain fitness while also having a good outlet for stress are sledge hammer exercises. By hitting a sledgehammer against a big rubber tire you will work your upper body in a way that it is most likely not used to being worked. This shock to the body will boost fitness.

183.   If you're using a personal trainer, pay them in advance. If you pay them now you're more likely to stick with the work since you won't want to have wasted that money. If you only pay the trainer at the session, you'll be more likely to give up since you won't have spent anything.

184.   You can build your run time by changing the way you breath. While running, when you inhale, breathe so that your belly rises. When you breath likes this you are ensuring that your lungs are fully inflating with oxygen. This will help you to run for a longer period of time.

185.   Keep your spine supple by doing spine mobilizing exercises. A supple spine is able to absorb impact better than one that is never exercised. Spine mobilizing exercises encourage the release of synovial fluid, which acts as a nourishing lubricant to your joints and also protects the discs in your back.

186.   If you injure one of your arms when pursuing your fitness goals, do not stop working out the other one. Research has discovered that people who only trained one arm for two weeks were able to increase their arm strength in the other arm by

around ten percent. This is because working out one arm also activates the fibers in the other arm.

187.   Proper exercise will require that you build up your stamina if you're overweight and relatively inactive. You can start to increase your stamina by working on your breathing techniques. When working out, you literally get "winded." Learn to take in more oxygen during your workout and you can increase your duration.

188.   Watch less television. Merely sitting and watching a few hours of tv shows means you are not up and around, which means that your body's metabolism is slowing down. Worse yet, chances of becoming obese increase with the amount of television that you watch. Instead of watching television, try taking a walk or playing a game.

189.   If you want to see immediate improvements in your bench press, try doing bench presses while looking at your dominant hand. Doing this will allow you to be able to lift more weight. However, you should never turn your head because this could cause injury. Instead, use your peripheral vision.

190.   Check your pulse to see if you need time off. If you had a strenuous workout, check your pulse the next morning. If it is still elevated at all, your body

is telling you it needs time to repair itself. Take it easy for a day.

191.   Do not be a single-machine user. Exercising in many different forms is the best way to do strength training, even if you want to focus on one part of your body. Overall strength and health is more important than getting bigger biceps, so try your best to be as diverse as possible.

192.   To help meet your goals of exercising regularly, invest in some home exercise equipment. If the equipment is right there, you won't be tempted to skip your exercise routine due to lack of time. Your motivation will be right there staring you in the face all evening and so you'll go do it.

193.   Sex makes an amazing weight loss tool. This is some of the most exciting and least work-like exercise you can do. Healthy sex will help you get fit and is a great way to include your partner in your pursuit for weight loss. You will get in shape and improve your relationship.

194.   To maximize your fitness routine and prevent injury, be sure to get rid of those old shoes. Shoes do not last forever, no matter how well you take care of them. They get worn down in certain areas and your foot leaves its own natural impression. In

order to provide the maximum amount of support and cushion, first check for wear to your shoe, otherwise, assume that heavy usage will get about one year out of your shoe and medium usage will get you two to three years, in general.

195.   Dedicating 30 minutes to working out every evening can actually go a long way. You can burn off a lot of the calories you consumed throughout the day by doing push ups and sit ups when you get home. You want to push yourself every time too, so that you get into shape as quickly as possible.

196.   You can build bigger biceps by bending your wrists slightly when you are doing arm curls with dumbbells. When your doing your arm curls, extend the wrists backwards slightly, and hold them like that. This slight change of movement will make your biceps work harder, thus, building bigger biceps.

197.   Starting a rigorous new workout program can be extremely daunting, especially if you plan to work with a trainer. If you are worried that you might not follow through with your commitment, pay your trainer the full amount up front. You will be less likely to skip workout sessions if you have already made a significant investment.

198.   In any kind of football, most people have trouble trying to shake their defender when going out to catch the ball. A good tip to do this is to stay as close as possible to him, then shorter your strides to allow you to cut in and out easier to catch the ball.

199.   When you are running up a hill, a great tip is to keep your head up with your eyes focused on the top of the hill. Doing this will open up your airways more than hunching your body forward. When your airways are open, your breathing is improved, which makes it easier to run up the hill.

200.   When working with heavy weights over your own body weight, you should always try and wear a weight belt. This helps keep your spine in line and in case something happens, it can prevent death or serious injury. This is essential with working out with weights that you might not be able to handle.

201.   With so many other exercises, you may forget to do sit ups. Sit ups help range of motion and have a positive effect on abdominal muscles, as they make your abs work longer and harder. Try to avoid anchoring you feet when doing sit ups-- that can strain your back.

202.   Smart fitness buffs do not subject themselves to long sets of crunches or sit-ups every day. The abdominal muscles that these exercises target are like any other set of muscles: They respond best when they get time to recover following a workout. The best results come from limiting ab workouts to two or three sessions a week.

203.   Hiring a qualified personal trainer has been proven to increase results. A recent study shows that those who had a personal trainer made significant improvements in fat mass, fat-free mass, strength and body mass, compared to those who did the same workouts, but on their own. Personal trainers can help with spotting, motivation and tips, on the exercises you are doing.

204.   Experiment with new exercises and new workouts to keep your fitness routine fresh. Once you have established a routine that works for you, you have to be on the lookout for boredom. Investigating and trying out new ways to exercise is not just fun; it prevents complacency and keep you dedicated to a fit, healthy lifestyle.

205.   When working out, do not forget about your trapezius muscle, a muscle that runs from the back of the neck to the upper part of your shoulders. Working on this muscle can help upper back and

neck pains. You can work on these muscles by holding dumbbells to your sides as you stand with your feet apart. Gradually bring up your shoulders and hold it that way for 8 seconds before releasing.

206.   Stay limber by stretching often, and if you are getting older, hold your stretches for longer periods of time. Your muscles will remain warm, strong and loose, and you will be able to workout more vigorously. Stretching can also help reduce or prevent soreness of the muscles and increases flexibility.

207.   Make sure to include fitness into every day of your life. Try to maximize every opportunity to burn calories. Choose the stairs over an escalator, or park your car in the last parking spot rather than the first. Use little breaks during the day get your blood pumping.

208.   If you're just starting out with exercise, start out slow. Don't jump in head first and try to run five miles without having exercised before. You can wind up injuring yourself and doing more harm than good. Instead start with a short walk and slowly increase the length and the speed. Before you know it you'll be running five miles without any problems.

209.   Increasing the amount of eggs one eats will increase the amount of protein the body takes in. It is very important for the development of fitness that the body has enough protein to build new muscle tissue. Choosing high protein foods will provide the materials the body needs.

210.   A great fitness tip is to follow a set order when working out. First, use dumbbells. Then, use barbells. Finally, use machines. You use this order because dumbbells focus on the smaller, stabilizer muscles that fatigue faster than the larger muscles. Once your smaller muscles are exhausted, move on to the machines to hit the larger muscle groups.

211.   Many people believe that changing from one grip width to another does not require any other adjustments to the weight that is being bench pressed. However, failure to make adjustments may cause unnecessary strain and stress of joints and muscles. Instead, a change in grip should be accompanied by a ten percent decrease in weight.

212.   Try exercising to reduce your overall cholesterol levels. Diet is enough to get them down to healthy levels, but you can get better and quicker results if you add exercising to your regimen. Generally, people who exercise have higher levels of HDL, or

good cholesterol and lower levels of LDL, or bad cholesterol, than those who only eat a healthier diet.

213.   Walk to lunch. If you work in an office environment, try walking to lunch at a place at least five minutes away. That way, after you've eaten and returned to work, you will have also done a nice 10 minute walk which can be healthy for your state of mind and body as well.

214.   If you want to speed up your swimming, build up the flexibility in your ankles. When you are in the water, your feet perform like flippers. So the more flexibility in your ankles, the quicker you can move through the water. A great way to build flexibility in your ankles is to lay on the floor, point your toes straight out, then flex them back towards you.

215.   You can get into your best physical shape when you do as much as you can to keep your body moving. A good policy is to always hand-deliver mail that has been sent to you erroneously. If the address is near you, take the time to do something good, and get in shape.

216.   Always pay attention to proper form when you are exercising your biceps. This is important because you can strain muscles in your arms. The proper form is to extend the wrist backwards

slightly and hold while you lift. When you release, slowly bring your wrist back to a straight resting position. This exertion will help to form the biceps that you desire in a safe manner.

217.   You need to find a workout that you actually enjoy doing if you really want to be able to stick to it. If you do not like what you are doing it will be very difficult to find the motivation to do it on a regular basis. A lot of people make the mistake of thinking fitness has to be boring and repetitive when it does not have to be.

218.   Weight lifters would do well to complement their workouts with a post workout drink. Studies have shown that significant gains can be achieved if a protein rich drink is ingested right after a workout. Your favorite protein shake would be just fine, or even a pint of chocolate milk has all the nutrients you need.

219.   Train with a friend to add focus and dedication to your fitness plan. Friends can not only be supportive, but can also add a bit of competition if they're on a more advanced fitness level than you. To really help, take it a step farther and plan meals around a diet plan that you share with your friend.

220.   Make sure you never workout when you are sick! That is, however, unless all your symptoms are above the neck. As a general rule, it is okay to workout if all your symptoms are restricted to the neck and above - this means your cardio vascular system will not be affected by the sickness.

221.   Give fitness enough time before you compare your results to your efforts. You should see results after a month of regular exercises. If you do not see any satisfying results after a month, you should rethink your routine or perhaps work out more. Do not stop exercising because you do not see results after one week only.

222.   A great fitness tip for basketball players is to run through dribbling drills while wearing leather or canvas gloves. The heavier materials will force your hands to become more sensitive which will result in much better ball control when you take the gloves off. Many NBA use this technique to help their game.

223.   A good tip for fitness people who want to try to work out before work, is to wake up 20 minutes earlier for the first week, and just go for a brisk walk. This gets your body acclimatized to working out first thing in the morning and it will make it easier to make the transition.

224.   Increase your activity level by not taking the easy routes during your day. Everyone has difficulty squeezing workouts into a hectic schedule, so increase your movement during the course of your normal day. Instead of parking near the entrance of the store, park at the end of the lot and walk. Avoid elevators and take the stairs whenever you can.

225.   Don't push yourself too hard when you are working out. While pushing yourself to your limits can be a good thing, be aware of those limits. Build your strength and stamina up gradually. If you intend on exercising daily, pushing yourself too hard only serves to discourage and tire you out the next day.

226.   Fitness takes discipline, so learn to kill your excuses before they start. Exercise routines typically falter because of laziness or disorganization. Buy an organizer and schedule out your exercise routine. This way, you'll stay on top of your routine and make sure that you're hitting all of your target areas on schedule.

227.   Once you have embarked on a new fitness routine, you may be tempted to overdo it. To build your strength and stamina, you should push yourself only slightly more each time you go into

your chosen activity. Stretching afterwards is key to ensuring you protect the muscles you are building.

228.   When planning your exercise routine, put in resistance first and the aerobic exercise last. When exercising glycogen is used first and then fat is used for energy. Glycogen will be used for the energy for resistance exercises. Doing aerobic exercise next will help you to burn more fat because the stored glycogen has already been used.

229.   Training for a marathon can be no easy feat. Try setting small goals to achieve each week that eventually lead up to being able to run or walk a 5k marathon. For some, walking that distance takes little effort, but for others it can feel like climbing Mount Everest. Take small walks or runs each day and push yourself to make it further and further each week.

230.   For your first day of working out, start slowly. Make sure you start with lower weights and gradually work your way up to bigger weights. If you don't do this, then the next morning you will be extremely sore and you can possibly damage part of your muscles or tissue.

231.   After a particularly strenuous workout of a muscle group, you can help your body to recover

from the stress by performing a lightly targeted workout of the affected muscles one day after. By gently engaging the muscle, you are helping it to repair itself faster by enabling your body to more efficiently deliver nutrients and blood to the area.

232.   You can make your legs much stronger by performing your standard leg crunches in reverse. This causes whichever leg you have in the front to get a great full muscle workout. These crunches are almost exactly like the standard leg crunches, except you are not stepping forward, you are stepping backward.

233.   When you are doing crunches, hold your tongue on the roof of your mouth during the duration of the crunches. It may seem silly, but when you do this, your head will align properly during this exercise. Using this method, you will greatly lower the strain on your neck while performing crunches.

234.   Change the exercises around that you do often. By alternating exercises, you will avoid boredom and prevent your body from plateauing. Combine high intensity exercises like kick boxing with low or medium intensity exercises such as walking or jogging. Keeping it fresh will keep you interested as well as helping your body.

235.   If you want to become better at hitting a softball, you should try playing Foosball. Foosball, also called table soccer, is a table game in which a ball is moved by controlling rods that are attached to player figurines. Playing Foosball on a regular basis will help you improve your hand-eye coordination, which will greatly assist you in hitting a softball.

236.   If you want to improve your putting when playing golf, a great tip is to aim high on breaks. Try to double where you think the break will be. This will allow you to get a lot closer to being accurate on your shot. Once you get used to doing this, you will see a noticeable difference in your putting.

237.   In order to increase strength, try lifting light weights fast. By lifting a lighter weight fast your muscles will generate greater force than if you were lifting a heavier weight slowly. To get the most out of this type of explosive training, select a weight that is 40 to 60 percent of your one rep maximum, and perform 8 sets of 3 repetitions. Each rep should be performed as fast as possible.

238.   After you workout it's important to do cool down exercises. Exercising causes your blood vessels to enlarge which makes your heart work harder to maintain your stamina during a workout.

Cool down exercises help your body to gradually return to it's normal functioning state and prevent unnecessary cardiovascular strain.

239.   Whenever you begin any fitness routine, it is best that you schedule an appointment to see your doctor. Your doctor can tell you things that you need to be aware of and what you need to do, and what your limits should be when exercising. Listening to what your doctor has to say is a good idea even if you're already close to your fitness goals.

240.   When you are weight lifting to increase fitness, it is always preferable to use free weights, not machines. This is because the free weights will allow you to build up the supporting muscles around the major muscle groups. Machines, instead, focus on very specific areas. You will see an increase in the amount of weight you can lift on the machine, but not as much strength as if you used free weights.

241.   In order to improve fitness levels when biking, try cycling with just one leg. The benefit of this is that you are able to focus on the important part of your leg stroke, that being the even distribution of workload among all of your leg muscles. This trains your leg for the upstroke and allows the minor, smaller muscles to get a greater workout.

242.   A great way to get fit is to invest in a bike. Riding a bike is a great way to get out and enjoy the outdoors. You can also burn a fair amount of calories. You can even ride your bike to take care of your errands.

243.   Try to work out in the morning. Why? Anything can happen to you during the day that makes you tired, stressed and flat out reluctant to exercise. By starting your day with exercise, you get it out of the way and it's done. You can go on with the rest of your day knowing you've already done something good for your body.

244.   When working out, is it important that you drink plenty of water. Drinking water while working out will maintain proper hydration, which is vital during any heavy exercising. Being hydrated will help you to work out harder and you will be able to exercise for a longer period of time. Always keep a water bottle with you and just keep drinking!

245.   A quick way to workout your leg muscles is to do squats. Simply hold your arms out, pointing forward away from your body, and crouch down with your legs. Then stand back up. Do this about ten times for three sets each. The stronger your legs get, the easier it will be to do them.

246. Have a timer handy when doing exercises at home. When using an exercise ball it is helpful to time each exercise so you know how long you are in each position. Holding each position for a specified length of time helps you build muscles and reach your fitness goals.

247. The intensity an individual puts into their own exercise activities will determine how effective they are at increasing fitness. The more one pushes their body during exercise the more it will grow. One needs to give a hundred percent to truly test themselves and challenge their bodies limits, expanding them at the same time.

248. It's important to start encouraging your children to exercise at an early age. It's better to get them into the habit right away rather than waiting until they are older. When they're older, they have to unlearn any lazy habits they have. It's much easier to get them to like exercising when they're little.

249. Do not be a single-machine user. Exercising in many different forms is the best way to do strength training, even if you want to focus on one part of your body. Overall strength and health is more important than getting bigger biceps, so try your best to be as diverse as possible.

250.   To get a progressive weigh-lifting program going, you should concentrate on increasing the absolute total weight you lift in each workout. The total weight comes from the weight you lift, times your number of reps, times your number of sets. You can increase total weight by adding to any of these three variables.

251.   While fitness should push our bodies, it is important though that you not push yourself too hard. By trying to exceed your body's capabilities, you are not doing yourself any favors; in fact, you may be causing yourself injury. For instance, when stretching, you should push yourself enough that you feel tension in the muscle, but not so far that you feel pain.

252.   In order to achieve a physically fit body, it is important that you know how to repair you muscles fast. If this is done efficiently, you can be able to workout your muscles as soon as they recover. Researchers found a fast way to repair muscles, and this is done by doing light exercises on the same muscles the following day.

253.   Having a rest day is important for your body and your state of mind when you are constantly being active and working out. Take one day a week

to just relax and gather yourself for another week of training. Be sure to stick to your diet in the meantime though.

254.   Always protect your neck when doing crunches. If you perform crunches incorrectly, you could hurt, strain, and even damage ligaments or muscle in your neck. Instead of using your neck to pull your body when doing crunches, you can put your tongue to the roof of your mouth in order to better align your head and neck.

255.   Karate can be a great way to improve your fitness. The belt tests make sure you always have a set of skills to learn and a goal to work towards. At some schools you may be able to train with the whole family. Not only will you be getting fit, but you'll also be building confidence.

256.   When working out, make sure you take your time and focus on doing any and all exercises properly. Even if you can't do as many or goes as long as you could if you were using short cuts, you'll get much better results by doing fewer perfect form exercises. Not to mention that by using short cuts or improper form you could end up injuring yourself

257. Do not let yourself be put off by the weather. The weather in no excuse not to work out. If you mean to jog outside and you find that it is raining, work around that. You can still get out and walk in a light drizzle. If the weather is terrible, find an alternative inside.

258. A good tip to help you lose weight is to exercise moderately. A lot of people make the mistake of going too hard at first. They'll do over two hours of cardio in one session and pretty soon they'll burn themselves out. It's best to go with a more moderate workout routine.

259. An easy way to work out your abs while doing any other activity is to hold in or flex your ab muscles. Doing this move on its own can, sometimes, be equivalent to doing a sit up. Doing it while working out or even just walking, helps strengthen the ab muscles and improves posture, since it is strengthening your core muscles.

260. If you want to build better abs, don't workout your abs daily. Although they can recover much quicker than other muscles, psychologically they are no different than other muscles. You will get better results if you take time between ab workouts. Try to exercise them only about two or three days in a week.

261. You should always work out with a partner. This is because they will give you motivation to actually go to the gym regularly. It is also important to bring them because they will spot you on things like a bench press so you do not end up hurting yourself.

262. You can't expect to see results right away, remember that. You have to stay focused and dedicated to your plan and a big part of that is your mentality. You can't expect to have abs in 2 weeks when this is your first time trying to get into shape, it takes months to get that lean body you are searching for.

263. Dreading and avoiding a certain type of exercise? That's all the more reason to push yourself to start it, and continue doing it. Reluctance to perform the exercise, is almost a surefire indicator that you are weak in that particular area - all the more reason to get started and overcome your reluctance.

264. If you are about to start a new fitness regime and have not exercised before or in a long time, or have a medical condition of some sort that might be exacerbated by exercise, it is a good idea to see your doctor before you begin a program. Getting a

medical check up will help ensure that you choose the most beneficial exercise program for yourself.

265.   The best way to build up your forehand strength for use with sports like tennis and racquetball is to do exercises with a crumpled newspaper. To do this properly, lay the paper flat on a surface. Start at a corner and crumple it into a ball shape with your dominant hand for about 30 seconds. Do the exact same with the other hand.

266.   If you have a dead tree on your property and are thinking of having a service remove it for you, you should reconsider. If you cut up the tree yourself with an axe or even a chainsaw, and then chop the logs to firewood with an axe, you will give yourself many great workouts and save on your fuel bill too!

267.   To get the best quality curls or shoulder presses, only exercise one arm at a time. Do one set with your right arm, then follow it up with an identical set with your left. By separating the two, you are more likely to see quality results than by doing the sets simultaneously.

268.   Do at least forty minutes of high-intensity aerobics a week to stay healthy. Studies have shown that people who work out are less likely to become ill, but if you only want to do the minimum, opt for

aerobics. People who performed two aerobics classes a week got sick much less often than those who don't exercise at all.

269.   A great tip to help you get fit is to not overlook the effectiveness of simple body weight exercises. Push ups, pullups, sit ups, and squats with only your body weight are very good exercises that are often overlooked. You can do them anywhere because you don't need any equipment.

270.   You need to decide exactly what you want, and go after it. Make a fitness goal and have no doubt that this is what you want to do. Once you have your mind made up, it will be less of a struggle because you will be determined to see it through.

271.   To get the best results from a workout that is largely comprised of walking, add some sprints into your regular walks. Running is one of the best full-body workouts available, but if you are not up to running long distances yet, then you can still get your heart pumping and give your metabolism a boost by alternating walking with 30-second sprints.

272.   When working be wary of the kinds of exercises you are doing in relation to the kind of body you are hoping to maintain. Some exercises are most helpful to people who are trying to burn fat. Some

are most helpful to those trying to build lean muscle. Some are best for those trying to build bulkier muscle. Be aware of what the exercises you are doing focus on.

273.   Do not weight train two days in a row. When exercising your muscles, be careful about working particular muscle groups too often and too much. After weight training, allow your muscles at least 48 hours to recover. Anything more does more harm than good. You won't see any favorable results.

274.   In order to maximize your fitness routine, be sure that you incorporate low fat milk into your diet. All of the commercials you saw growing up were right, milk is great for your body. Along with a well balanced diet, it will assist in muscle growth, and keeping your body fat content down.

275.   Making exercise fun is one of the best ways to stay fit. Dragging yourself to the gym or engaging in any other activities you don't enjoy will discourage you from working out more. Find something physically demanding that you enjoy. Joining a local sports team is a great way to make friends, have fun, and stay in shape.

276.   When strength training or working with weights, try to keep your daily workout under 60 minutes.

After an hour, your body responds to strength-building exercises by producing excessive amounts of cortisol. This hormone can block the production of testosterone and may actually impair the body's ability to build and maintain muscle.

277.   Don't regard fitness clothing shopping as trying to select something for the catwalk. You need to focus on fit and function when looking for clothes. Make sure they are comfortable and well-fitted pieces that go with everything. Try sticking to the neutrals like black, white, and gray since they accomplish that.

278.   Try doing dips that use double the energy to give your triceps a more effective workout during your routine. Start by doing your dips like you usually would, but with your elbows turned inward and keeping your body straightened. Then lean forward and force them outward to focus on your chest muscles.

279.   If you are a student, join a sports team of your choice. Sports teams are great to instill discipline and will help you to get in shape quickly and efficiently. The constant exercises and running that you will do during practice will help you to get to your weight goal desired.

280.   A good fitness tip is to start performing shoulder shrugs. Shoulder shrugs are a great way to beef up your trapezoid muscles. Your trapezoid muscles are located on your collarbone. Shoulder shrugs are very easy to perform but as always, it's not a good idea to lift more weight than you can handle.

281.   If you want your kids to get more exercise, try making it a competition. Buy everyone in your family a pedometer. Each day mark down how many steps each person has walked. At the end of the week, tally the totals up and see who the winner is. Come up with a good prize for the winner - a new toy, an extra desert, or getting to choose dinner for the night.

282.   Add your workout to your daily schedule, and follow it. Many people say that they do not have the time to exercise, but if you add it to your calendar and try it out, you will probably find that you still accomplished everything else you had to do. Lose the excuse, and get to work!

283.   Go with a friend. Studies have shown that taking someone along with you to a gym is likely to not only increase the amount of time you stay, but also the intensity of your workout. Some gyms offer

discounts when multiple people register together, so take advantage of this and bring someone along!

284. Focus on your workout. As long as you are making the time for fitness, make the most of your time by really focusing on your workout. If you are going at a pace at which you can comfortably chat on the phone or read a book, you are cheating yourself out of results. Really push yourself during your workout and save the leisure activities for later.

285. Believe it or not, what you wear during a workout routine is very important. Wearing heavy clothing is not advised because it can make you sweat more and cause dehydration. To give the proper support to your breasts during exercise, wearing a sports bra is recommended.

286. Protein shakes and other weightlifting supplements are most effective when consumed immediately after a workout. Fitness enthusiasts who concentrate their exercise routines on building muscle mass will do lots of weightlifting and also likely use protein shakes to fuel their workouts. Research has found that the best time to fuel up is directly following exercise, rather than hours after finishing or before starting.

287.   If you are trying to focus on losing belly fat, do not work on your abs. Although you will gain muscle, you are not losing fat. It is okay to do sit ups and crunches, but incorporate more aerobic exercises into your routine in order to lose unwanted belly fat.

288.   At the end of your exhaustive workout session, rather than reaching for a sports drink or water, try chocolate milk. Chocolate milk has been shown to hydrate as well as water but speeds the recovery time of athletes in training. You will be able to return to another workout session faster than if you had chosen a different beverage.

289.   Take some time out of your workout to focus specifically on your trouble areas. Doing this will make sure that you give special attention to the things you need to work on, and the extra time will translate to better results. Trouble areas won't be trouble too long if you give them special consideration.

290.   To help you include exercise into a tight schedule, you should walk whenever possible. That could mean taking the stairs instead of the elevator at the office or parking at the back of a large lot to give you a brisk brief walk to the store. When it comes to working out, every little bit counts.

291.   Cut down on your workout time and work on your weaknesses by using the same weight for your entire workout. To determine what that weight should be, try focusing on your weakest exercise and then pick a weight that you can lift between 6 and 8 times in a single circuit.

292.   If you want to run or walk your way to fitness, be sure to take safety precautions to keep yourself and others safe. Try running in the opposite direction of traffic so you can see oncoming cars in busy traffic. It is also safer to run or walk during the day so you can be seen more easily. Having a partner also adds to safety. But, try moving in a single-file line to avoid large groups that could endanger members.

293.   Practice your running form. Your feet should always hit the ground directly under your body, not in front of, or behind you. Your toes should be the way you propel yourself forward, not the ball of your foot or the heel. Getting running form correct is the best way to maximize your running potential.

294.   Building forearm strength is easier than you might know and can be done almost anywhere. When you are finished with your newspaper, save a few sheets for working out. Place a sheet from the

paper on a table or other flat surface. Simply start at one corner and crumple it into your hand, pulling the paper in as you go. Try to make this take about 30 seconds for maximum effect. Do this with both hands.

295.   A great tip to help you get physically fit is to start playing tennis. There's no such thing as an overweight tennis player because of all the running they have to do back and forth on the court. You can play it competitively or you can just play against your friends.

296.   Prior to embarking on a weight lifting regimen with the goal of improving your arms, know exactly what you plan to achieve. If your goal is to have larger muscles, your plan should include heavy lifting. To tone and sculpt, do more repetitions with lighter weights.

297.   While lifting weights, squeeze your butt muscles together. By doing this, you are putting your body into a position that stabilizes your spine, thus reducing injuries or strains to your lower back. Make sure that as you are squeezing your butt muscles together that you are lifting the weights over your head.

298.   A great tip to build forearm strength for tennis players is to crumple up some newspaper. Start by laying a newspaper on a flat surface and from one corner, crumple it into a ball with your dominant hand for at least 30 seconds. This exercise isolates your forearm muscles and is a great way to work them out.

299.   Stepping classes are an especially great way for women to get fit. Stepping classes can shape up the thighs and butt, a region that's well-known for being important in feminine beauty! Other exercises such as body squats and lunges can also help to firm up these muscles as well. Trunk, core and thigh muscles are important to both genders, because they provide a majority of the body's lifting capability.

300.   The best thing you can do for fitness is to stop smoking. You will have more energy and better circulation when you quit. Very soon your lungs will clear and you will be exercising at optimum levels. On top of that, you will get better sleep and have better moods. Quitting smoking is the #1 way to improve your fitness levels.

301.   Health and fitness is psychological and not just physical, so do your best to... avoid the scales! Scales tend to frustrate people especially if they are

checking it every day and see no progress. Many don't realize that they are losing weight and trimming fat but gaining muscle at the same time so the progress isn't as noticeable in the beginning. It's recommended that you weigh yourself no more than twice a month. At the beginning and the middle of the month just to track things for your fitness routine.

302.   Whenever you are lifting weights that target your arms, it is generally a good idea to lift one arm at a time. Often times, one arm is stronger than the other and can do more of the work whenever you lift with both arms at the same time. Exercises which isolate your arms will ensure that both get a proper workout.

303.   Sometimes it can be hard for to maintain a daily exercise regimen, but here are a few quick tips to help you stick with it. 1) Set a daily alarm or daily reminder on your phone to encourage you to exercise, make it encouraging and positive. Remember, this is something you want to do! 2) Set the reminder for a time when you usually don't have anything pressing to do. Such as after you come home from work or right when you wake up or go to bed. 3) Remember, you can split your daily exercise to two 15 minute sessions. IT can

sometimes be easier to find 15 minutes than it to find 30, so perhaps set two alarms during the day.

304.   One way to stay healthy and fit when working out is to do all that you can to prevent neck injury. Never exert yourself without proper guidance and knowledge. Always use proper form when performing any type of strength building exercise. Be sure to stretch your neck properly before and after the workout.

305.   When it comes to exercise, don't take the "all or nothing" approach. It is much better to sneak in a little bit of exercise than to do nothing at all. Just a simple walk will help with your overall health. If you only have one day a week to commit to strength training, you will still see benefits.

306.   Dancing is a fun way to get fit! To dance in the comfort of your own home, find an open area such as a living room or basement. Turn on the radio or find some music on your computer that you would like to dance to. Listen to the beat and let your body move in any way or form that feels comfortable. Nobody's watching, so let loose and don't feel embarrassed!

307.   When doing crunches, make sure that your neck is properly protected. The neck can easily be

strained or hurt and cause major problems because of its location. You can easily align your neck by touching your tongue to the roof of your mouth. It straightens the alignment of your neck to prevent neck strain or injury.

308.   If you are going to use a bench, you should always test it first. If the bench is too hard, it may cause a misalignment in your spine that can weaken your arm. Test the bench by pushing a thumb into the padding. If you can feel the wood underneath the padding, find a better bench to use.

309.   If you are trying to flatten your stomach, a great tip is to be sure you work out your invisible abdominal muscles. These are the trasversus abdominis muscles, which are beneath your rectus abdominis. They flatten your waist when you suck in your stomach. In order to work this muscle out, try to pull in your belly button towards your spine. While breathing normally, hold this position for ten seconds.

310.   When you go to the gym for a weight workout, think small to large when it comes to your activities. Begin with with dumbbells and end with machine work. The smaller muscles you need to use with dumbbell work tend to tire more quickly than the larger muscle groups used in machines. Therefore,

end with the machines as your body will then need less from those smaller muscle groups.

311.　When you are doing crunches, push your tongue firmly against the roof of your mouth. Doing so forces you to straighten out your neck, preventing any chances of neck injury. This also helps to decrease neck fatigue, and allows you to increase the amount of crunches you are able to do in one sitting.

312.　A fun and effective way to help you get fit is to purchase a soccer ball to kick around. Playing soccer is one of the best sports for shaping up because there is so much running involved. You can just play with your friends if you don't want to play competitively.

313.　Those with asthma can safely exercise everyday if they stay hydrated. It's reported that dehydration may increase the likelihood of an asthma attack while exercising. A recent study found that those with exercise-induced asthma had a significant decrease in their lung function when dehydrated. The theory is that dehydration can cause a tightening of the lungs' airways.

314.　Switch up your workout routine so you don't get tired of exercise. You may find another workout you really enjoy more than another. This will also keep your focus on a variety of fitness techniques instead of doing the same thing daily. It's also better for your muscles and helps to develop them with different exercises.

315.   Stop making excuses for not working out. Schedule a block of time to workout tomorrow, even if it's only for 15 minutes. Tomorrow, schedule another block of time for the next day. Do this daily and eventually you won't need to make that appointment with yourself and your workout time will increase. Soon, exercise will just be part of a normal day.

316.   Fitness is more fun when you vary your workouts. By doing the same workout everyday or even a few times a week, your mind and body are bound to get bored quickly. If you vary your workouts several times a week, it not only gives your mind something to look forward to but it also gives your body a nice change. By doing different exercises, you are working different muscles each time, which in turn will result in maximum weight loss and a more toned body.